Fre

all about
echinacea &
goldenseal

LAUREL VUKOVIĆ

AVERY PUBLISHING GROUP
Garden City Park • New York

The information contained in this book is based upon the research and personal and professional experiences of the author. It is not intended as a substitute for consulting with your physician or other health care provider. Any attempt to diagnose and treat an illness should be done under the direction of a health care professional.

The publisher does not advocate the use of any particular health care protocol, but believes the information in this book should be available to the public. The publisher and author are not responsible for any adverse effects or consequences resulting from the use of any of the suggestions, preparations, or procedures discussed in this book. Should the reader have any questions concerning the appropriateness of any procedure or preparation mentioned, the author and the publisher strongly suggest consulting a professional health care advisor.

Series cover designer: Eric Macaluso
Cover image courtesy of Steven Foster Group, Inc.

Avery Publishing Group, Inc.
120 Old Broadway, Garden City Park, NY 11040
1-800-548-5757 or visit us at www.averypublishing.com

ISBN: 0-89529-937-2

Printed in the United States of America

10   9   8   7   6   5   4   3   2   1

Contents

Introduction

If I had to choose only one herb to keep in my medicine cabinet, it would be echinacea. I've been using herbs for more than twenty-five years and teaching and writing about them for almost a decade. Out of the more than three dozen medicinal herbs that I have at home, echinacea is the one that I reach for more often than any other. I've used it countless times to ward off colds and flus, to stave off urinary tract infections, and to heal infected wounds. For any type of infection, echinacea is my herb of choice. Not only is it a safe and gentle herb, but it is also remarkably effective for helping the immune system overcome infectious microorganisms. When taken at the first sign of illness, echinacea can even prevent a full-blown infection.

Natural compounds in echinacea stimulate the immune system to do what it is designed to do, only better. Essentially, echinacea provides a helping hand to the immune system. In contrast, prescription and over-the-counter drugs merely suppress symptoms and actually have been shown to prolong the course of an illness because they interfere with immune function. Our bodies have evolved with centuries of healing wisdom stored in our cells, and often the best thing we can do is support the natural process of healing, rather than overrule it. Echinacea does just that. It enhances many aspects of immune function and strengthens the immune system.

Goldenseal is another of my favorite healing herbs. It is a potent antimicrobial and has been proven to be effective against a wide variety of infectious microorganisms. I've seen goldenseal effectively treat bronchial infections, sinusitis, urinary tract infections, eye infections, and candidiasis. Together, echinacea and goldenseal make a powerful immune-boosting and infection-fighting team that is safer, less expensive, and often as effective as prescription antibiotics, without the harmful side effects. Of course, if you have any type of serious infectious disease, you should not attempt self-treatment and should consult with your health-care practitioner for guidance.

A strong immune system is more important in today's world than ever before. We are constantly bombarded with substances that tax our bodies and weaken our immunity, from poisonous chemicals in our air, water, and food to toxins created in our own bodies as by-products of emotional and physical stressors. Immune-deficiency diseases are on the rise, and diseases that were thought to be eradicated, such as tuberculosis, are making a frightening comeback. The antibiotic drugs that we have relied so heavily upon are turning out to have a serious backlash effect, creating supergerms for which we have no effective medical treatments.

The answer lies not in attempting to eradicate all infectious microbes, but in strengthening the immune system and using nontoxic antimicrobial herbs when necessary to fight trouble-causing microorganisms. Read on to learn more about how echinacea and goldenseal can help you do this.

1.

A Brief Guide to Your Immune System

Your immune system may be the most complex system of your body, and scientists are still uncovering new insights about how the organs, glands, and cells function to keep the body healthy. A basic knowledge of how your immune system works will help you better understand how echinacea and goldenseal can help you. Of course, you don't have to understand everything about the intricacies of your immune system for echinacea and goldenseal to be effective. This chapter presents an overview.

Q. How do germs get into my body in the first place?

A. There are many different avenues of entry. In general, your skin acts as an excellent protective barrier against harmful microorganisms, but cuts and wounds provide easy access. Infectious organisms are also able to enter into the interior of the body through the mucous membranes of the mouth, throat, lungs, intestinal tract, and genitourinary tract. Bacteria, viruses, fungi, and protozoa thrive in a warm, dark, moist environment—the interior of the body is a perfect place for them to set up housekeeping. Fortunately, most of the time, a healthy immune system keeps them in check.

Q. How does my immune system protect me from disease?

A. The primary job of the immune system is to protect the body against infectious microorganisms and to prevent the development of cancer. Your immune system is constantly on patrol, checking cells for evidence of infection and looking for cells that show cancerous changes. The immune system offers two types of protection against disease: nonspecific resistance to disease and specific resistance to disease (also known as immunity).

Q. Can you explain nonspecific resistance to disease?

A. Nonspecific defensive responses are the body's first response to invading microorganisms. They include the natural barriers provided by healthy skin and mucous membranes, antimicrobial chemicals, phagocytosis, natural killer cells, inflammation, and fever. All nonspecific defenses protect the body against a variety of pathogens and foreign substances. Here's how nonspecific defense works: If infectious microorganisms penetrate the barrier provided by the skin and mucous membranes, antimicrobial chemicals in the blood, such as *interferons* and *complement fractions*, are waiting as a second line of defense. If these fail, the next immune players brought into action include *natural killer cells*, which kill a wide variety of infectious microorganisms and tumor cells, and *phagocytes*, white blood cells that engulf and destroy infected and damaged cells.

In addition, inflammation and fever help to protect the body. When microorganisms invade the body, they damage tissues, causing inflammation. Inflammation promotes the disposal of toxins and microorganisms at the site of the injury and prevents the spread of infection. With the extra blood flow that occurs with inflammation, large numbers of white blood cells flood the affected area. They destroy the invaders, and in many cases, this is enough to defeat the infection. Fever also helps the body overcome infection by inhibiting the growth of microbes and enhancing the effect of interferon, the body's natural virus-fighting chemical.

Q. What is specific resistance to disease?

A. This refers to immunity, or the ability of the body to defend itself against specific antigens—substances that the immune system recognizes as foreign and that provoke an immune response. There are two types of immune responses involved in specific resistance to disease: cell-mediated immune responses, and antibody-mediated immune responses.

Q. What is cell-mediated immunity?

A. Cell-mediated immunity begins when the body's T cells (a type of white blood cell) recognize an antigen (foreign invader). The T cells begin a complex process of enlarging, multiplying, and forming highly specialized cells to mount an attack against the invader. This type of immune activity is important for overcoming infection by such microorganisms as yeast, fungi, parasites, viruses, and moldlike bacteria. Chronic or recurring infections, such as candidiasis and herpes, indicate that cell-mediated immunity is not functioning optimally. In addition, cell-mediated immunity protects the body against allergies, autoimmune diseases such as rheumatoid arthritis, and cancer.

Q. What is antibody-mediated immunity?

A. In the presence of an antigen, B cells (a specialized type of white blood cell) in the lymph nodes and spleen are activated and produce plasma cells, which secrete antibodies that travel to the site of the invasion through the lymph and blood. These antibodies combine with the antigen and disable it. Specialized B cells remember any antigen that has triggered an immune response, as do the T cells, thus providing long-term immunity to that particular antigen.

Q. Where exactly is my immune system in my body?

A. It's not possible to pinpoint an exact location

because there are many different components, and your immune system is spread throughout your body. The thymus gland (found at the base of the neck), spleen (located just under the rib cage on the left side of the body), bone marrow, and a large network of lymph nodes (including the tonsils) make up the basic structure of the immune system. Hundreds of lymph nodes are scattered throughout the body, and are concentrated primarily in the armpits, neck, groin, abdomen, and chest.

The thymus gland, spleen, and bone marrow manufacture a variety of white blood cells, including neutrophils, lymphocytes, eosinophils, basophils, and monocytes. These almost colorless cells circulate throughout the blood and lymph fluid, protecting the body from invading microorganisms. In addition, the immune system is composed of specialized immune cells called macrophages and mast cells, which are found not just in the bloodstream but throughout the body, and special compounds that stimulate white blood cells to destroy cancer cells and cells infected by microorganisms. These compounds include interferon, interleukin II, and complement fractions. Interferon is made by the T cells, interleukins are made by both T cells and macrophages, and complement fractions are produced in the liver and spleen.

Q. What role does the thymus gland play in immunity?

A. Although it is often ignored, the thymus gland is the most important gland of the immune system and is responsible for a number of immune-related functions. It produces T cells, the white blood cells in charge of cell-mediated immunity, and also releases several hormones that regulate immune function. Low levels of thymus hormones are found in the elderly, cancer and AIDS patients, and people who are under a great deal of stress. To a large extent, you are only as healthy as your thymus gland. If you suffer from frequent or chronic infections, you most likely have impaired thymus function.

Q. What role does the spleen play in immunity?

A. The spleen nestles in the upper left abdomen just behind the lower ribs and is about the size of your fist. It is the largest lymphatic organ, and primarily produces white blood cells, cleanses the blood of bacteria and cellular debris, and destroys worn-out red blood cells. In addition, the spleen releases compounds that enhance immune activity.

Q. What is lymph?

A. Lymph is a clear, colorless fluid that bathes and cleanses all of the cells of your body. It flows through the lymphatic system, a network of porous lymphatic vessels similar to arteries that runs parallel to the circulatory system. Lymph passes into and out of the bloodstream through permeable membranes, bringing nutrients to cells and carrying away waste products. This cellular debris is filtered through the lymph nodes, as well as the tonsils, adenoids, appendix, spleen, and Peyer's patches (small masses of lymphatic tissue in the small intestine).

Q. What role does the lymphatic system play in immune function?

A. Anytime you have an active infection, the lymph nodes closest to the affected area swell to contain the toxins. For example, you've probably noticed tender, swollen lymph nodes under your jaw when you've had a sore throat. As lymph is filtered through the lymph nodes, bacteria and other trouble-causing microorganisms are attacked and consumed by white blood cells. Macrophages are the cells that cleanse the lymph. These large white blood cells, sometimes referred to as "big eaters," engulf and destroy harmful microorganisms, cancer cells, and cellular debris. The lymph nodes also contain B cells, a type of white blood cell that initiates the production of antibodies in response to infectious microorganisms. When the infection has been overcome, the lymph nodes return to normal, which is about the size of a small pea.

Q. What role do the various types of white blood cells play in immune functioning?

A. The primary function of white blood cells is to protect the body against pathogens. Neutrophils play an important role in preventing bacterial infection. They engulf and destroy bacteria, cellular debris, and cancer cells. Lymphocytes are a large family of white blood cells, and include T cells, B cells, and natural killer cells. T cells are produced in the thymus gland, and circulate throughout the blood and lymph. They are involved in many immune functions, including cell-mediated immunity. There are several different types of T cells, including helper T cells, which support the functioning of other white blood cells; suppressor T cells, which inhibit the activity of other white blood cells; and cytotoxic T cells (also known as killer T cells), which destroy cancer cells and virus-infected cells. B cells are responsible for producing antibodies to specific antigens, and natural killer cells destroy infected and cancerous cells. Eosinophils and basophils release compounds that break down antigen-antibody complexes and regulate inflammatory and allergic responses. Monocytes are large white blood cells that clean up cellular debris after an infection. Macrophages are immune cells that reside in tissues such as the lymph nodes, liver, and spleen.

Q. How exactly does echinacea affect my white blood cells?

A. Echinacea stimulates white blood cell production and activity. Polysaccharides, immune stimulating substances found in echinacea, bind to receptors on the surface of white blood cells and activate them. The white blood cells that have been found to be most affected by echinacea are T cells, macrophages, and natural killer cells.

Q. I'm not sure if my immune system is functioning up to par. How can I tell?

A. If you catch colds easily or come down with more than two colds per year, your immune system is not functioning as well as it could be. Other symptoms of poor immune function include cuts or wounds that are slow to heal; chronic viral, fungal, or yeast infections, such as athlete's foot, herpes, or candidiasis; sore or swollen lymph glands; chronic allergies; and any type of recurring infection, such as a urinary tract infection or respiratory infection. Excessive fatigue is another symptom that should alert you to the possibility that your immune system is not functioning up to par.

Q. How can I keep my immune system healthy?

A. An overall healthful lifestyle can do much to ensure that your immune system is operating at peak efficiency. Avoid smoking, drugs, and alcohol.

Eat a diet of fresh, natural foods, emphasizing organically grown and minimally processed foods. Fresh fruits and vegetables, in particular, are rich sources of cell-protecting nutrients—strive for at least five servings daily. Avoid hydrogenated, poly-unsaturated, and saturated fats, and foods treated with chemicals and hormones, all of which create cell damage. Minimize sweets, including honey, maple syrup, and all concentrated sweeteners. All types of sugars have been shown to impair immune functioning. It's a good idea to take a high-potency multivitamin/multimineral supplement. Nutritional deficiencies, especially of the B-complex vitamins and the cell-protecting nutrients vitamins A, C, and E, selenium, and zinc are associated with depressed immune function.

Regular daily exercise not only improves your general health, but specifically strengthens the immune system. But overdoing exercise—more than about an hour a day of aerobic activity—has been shown to actually impair immune functioning. Emotional stress as well as physical stress has a direct negative effect on the immune system. Take time every day to relax and unwind, make sure to get sufficient sleep, and cultivate a positive attitude towards life. In general, happy people are healthier people!

2.

The Healing Properties of Echinacea

Echinacea (pronounced eck-uh-*nay*-sha) ranks as one of the most popular medicinal herbs in the United States and Europe, and for good reason. This gentle, safe herb is a powerful ally that protects the body against all types of infectious diseases, without any harmful side effects. More than 400 scientific studies have proven the effectiveness of echinacea in treating infectious diseases. In this chapter, you'll learn about how echinacea came to be so popular, and what it can do for you.

Q. What is echinacea?

A. Echinacea is a member of the *Compositae* family, a large botanical family that includes daisies, marigolds, and dandelions. A one- to four-foot tall perennial, echinacea is a favorite of gardeners. It looks a lot like black-eyed Susan, with beautiful purple petals radiating outward from dark cone-shaped centers. (Some less common varieties of echinacea have pink, white, or yellow petals.) The genus *Echinacea* was named in 1794 by the botanist Moench. The name comes from the Greek word *echinos*, meaning sea urchin or hedgehog—an apt description of the prickly cone at the center of the echinacea flower.

Echinacea is native to the plains of the United States and grows wild nowhere else in the world except for a few places in southern Canada. Of the nine different echinacea species that are indigenous to the United States, three have been used histori-cally and have been clinically studied in both the United States and in Europe: *Echinacea purpurea* (purple coneflower), *Echinacea angustifolia* (narrow-leaved coneflower), and *Echinacea pallida* (pale cone-flower). All parts of echinacea are used medicinal-ly—the flower head, leaves, stem, and root.

Q. Why should I be interested in echinacea?

A. If you're interested in staying healthy, echinacea deserves a prominent place in your medicine cabinet. Every day, we all encounter a variety of potentially harmful microorganisms—viruses, bacteria, fungi, and protozoa—that are trying to penetrate our defenses. Our immune systems do their best to protect us, but sometimes these troublemaking organisms slip through, causing diseases such as colds, flus, bronchitis, staph infections, yeast infections, and strep throat. You've most likely suffered through first-hand experience with one or more of these common ailments. The prescription and over-the-counter medicines that are conventionally prescribed to treat these diseases often are toxic, cause unpleasant side effects, and are expensive.

Echinacea is a powerful, safe, and inexpensive alternative. Not only does it help your body fight off invading microorganisms, but it works in harmony with your immune system to keep you healthy. Echinacea can be taken for a few days to knock out a cold or flu, or it can be taken over a period of a few months to strengthen your overall immunity. Because it is one of the most powerful natural immune-boosting herbs available, echinacea has become one of the most popular herbs in the United States and Europe.

Q. How long has echinacea been used as a healing herb?

A. Archeologists have found evidence of echinacea in American Indian sites dating back to the 1600s. Plants were the Native American's primary form of medicine, and echinacea was the favorite herb of the Plains Indians. They used it extensively to treat all types of infections, including colds, coughs, sore throats, blood poisoning, gonorrhea, wounds, smallpox, and snakebites. They used echinacea in a variety of ways, making it into poultices and teas, and often simply sucked on a piece of the root as a convenient way of taking the herb.

The Native Americans generously shared their knowledge of echinacea's healing properties with the European settlers, who quickly adopted the plant. In 1870, Dr. H. C. F. Meyer, a German physician in Pawnee City, Nebraska, concocted a patented herbal medicine made with echinacea. He named it "Meyer's Blood Purifier" and claimed it as a cure-all for a variety of ailments, including snakebite. He believed so strongly in the healing properties of echinacea that in 1887, he tried to promote it to two of the most prominent Eclectic physicians of the time, Dr. John Uri Lloyd (a professor at the Eclectic Medical Institute in Cincinnati and later president of the American Pharmaceutical Association) and Dr. John King (author of *King's American Dispensatory*). To prove the efficacy of echinacea, he offered to let himself be bitten by a rattlesnake in the presence of the doctors and to treat himself only with echinacea. The doctors declined his offer, surmising that he was a quack.

Q. So how did echinacea come to be accepted as a legitimate herbal remedy?

A. Meyer persisted and persuaded King to at least give echinacea a try. Although he didn't opt for the snakebite experiment, King did try echinacea for a variety of illnesses and was convinced of the herb's healing properties after using it successfully to treat bee stings, sinusitis, and infant cholera. John Uri Lloyd also reversed his previously negative position on echinacea, proclaiming the herb useful for treating poisonous bites and stings, wounds, gangrene, malaria, blood poisoning, and the infectious diseases that were so devastating at that time— diphtheria, scarlet fever, influenza, meningitis, measles, and chickenpox.

The Lloyd family pharmaceutical company began marketing echinacea formulations, and the herb quickly became a favorite of both Eclectic and conventional physicians. At that time, *Echinacea angustifolia* was believed to be the most potent form of echinacea. Preparations of echinacea were a common remedy in home medicine chests from the 1890s until the advent of antibiotics in the 1930s.

Q. Who were the Eclectic physicians?

A. From the mid-1800s through the 1930s, there were two primary schools of medicine practiced in the United States. The orthodox physicians (known as "regulars") practiced conventional medicine, while the Eclectics relied heavily on the use of herbs for healing, much as naturopathic physicians do today. With the discovery of pharmaceutical antibiotics, which appeared to work miracles, orthodox medicine took over in the United States and edged out the Eclectics. It's only been in recent years that a more holistic approach to health has emerged, and with it, a resurgence of interest in herbal medicine.

Q. How did echinacea manage to survive the opposition of orthodox physicians to herbal medicine?

A. Fortunately, herbal medicine never took a beating in Europe the way it did in the United States. European doctors have always regarded herbs as legitimate medical treatments, and herbal products are commonly sold in European pharmacies. Echinacea was introduced to Europe sometime in the early 1900s. In 1932, a German scientist named Gerhard Madaus proved that the fresh-pressed juice from *Echinacea purpurea* flowers had potent immune-strengthening properties. In the ensuing years, approximately 400 scientific studies have proven the powerful positive effects that echinacea has on the immune system. With these studies, *E. purpurea* became as respected as *E. angustifolia* among herbal practitioners. Since the 1930s, European markets have bought more than 50,000 pounds of echinacea from the United States each year. Another European, the naturopathic doctor Alfred Vogel, was also introduced to echinacea by a Native American chief. Vogel also recognized that freshly prepared echinacea was more potent than the dried herb, and he helped spread the word about this remarkable plant.

Q. Why is echinacea so popular now?

A. A renaissance of interest in echinacea was sparked in about 1980, when immune disorders such as candidiasis, chronic fatigue syndrome, and acquired immunodeficiency syndrome (AIDS) began to appear. With medical science having so little to offer, people suffering from these and other chronic immune diseases began turning to alternative treatments. The consumer-driven trend toward natural medicine, including herbal medicine, has also fueled echinacea's popularity. The long history of echinacea as a safe infection-fighting herb and the decades of scientific support that the Europeans have amassed attesting to the efficacy of echinacea make it a logical choice for an immune-enhancing herbal medicine.

Q. What exactly does echinacea do?

A. Echinacea protects your body against invading microorganisms in a number of ways. It stimulates the activity of leukocytes, white blood cells that fight infection, and T lymphocytes (also known as T cells). It also has action similar to interferon, a chemical produced by the body that fights viruses. At the same time, echinacea increases the activity of macrophages, white blood cells that devour harmful microorganisms and infected and damaged cells.

In addition to all of the above, echinacea appears to have mild antibiotic properties. And if microbes such as viruses sneak past your defenses, echinacea can still help. It prevents viruses from gaining a foothold on cell surfaces by blocking virus receptors on cells, and prevents microbes from penetrating tissues. It also speeds wound healing by stimulating new, healthy cell growth.

Q. What is in echinacea that makes it so powerful as an immune stimulant?

A. It's important to understand that while echinacea is one of the most popular and widely used herbal medicines in the United States and Europe, there is still much to be learned about how it actually works. Researchers differ in their opinions about the most valuable constituents, and to confuse the matter further, different varieties of echinacea contain different constituents. With these considerations in mind, here is a brief attempt to explain the active compounds found in echinacea.

Echinacea contains a wide variety of immune-enhancing natural chemicals, all of which seem to work together to strengthen immunity. The major important medicinal constituents identified in the plant thus far are *polysaccharides*, *flavonoids* (a group of beneficial compounds found in plants), *caffeic acid derivatives*, *essential oils*, *polyacetylenes*, and *alkylamides*. Many researchers consider polysaccharides to be the primary immune-enhancing ingredient in echinacea. Polysaccharides are large, complex, water-soluble, sugar molecules found in plants and mushrooms. Scientists theorize that polysaccharides resemble compounds in the cell walls of bacteria and that this case of mistaken identity rouses the immune system into action. But other researchers believe that while the polysaccharides in echinacea do demonstrate strong activity, they may be broken down in the digestive tract before they have a chance to be absorbed into the bloodstream.

Echinacoside and cichoric acid are both derived from caffeic acid (an immune-enhancing phytochemical) and are also water-soluble components of echinacea. Echinacoside is a natural antibiotic and has been used as a marker for standardizing some echinacea formulas. But echinacoside has only mild antibiotic activity and has not been shown to actually have immune-enhancing activity. However, in laboratory tests, researchers have found that cichoric acid from echinacea stimulates the activity of macrophages.

Other researchers believe that alkylamides and polyacetylenes, the fat-soluble components of echinacea, are primarily responsible for the plant's immune-strengthening benefits. Alkylamides are uncommon plant constituents, and give echinacea its unique tongue-tingling sensation. They are found in higher concentrations in *E. purpurea* and *E. angustifolia*, and low concentrations in *E. pallida*. However, *E. pallida* contains polyacetylenes, also considered to have immune-enhancing properties.

Q. If scientists don't know how echinacea works, how do I know that it has value?

A. It's not unusual that scientists are not united in agreeing about the way in which echinacea works. Isolating the active constituents of a plant is a painstaking process that involves a great deal of research. It's not easy to determine which compounds have medicinal action, and the task is made more difficult because laboratory tests performed on blood samples are not always an accurate reflection of what happens in the body. For example, the medicinal compounds found in plants may work together to create a healing effect, and if they are taken as separate entities, they may not have the same effect.

What we do know is that many studies have proven that echinacea improves immune function. Not knowing exactly *how* it strengthens immunity does not negate the positive benefits of this remarkable herb.

Q. What are the most common uses for echinacea?

A. Echinacea is most commonly used for treating all types of general infections. It is perhaps best known for preventing and treating colds and flus, and is excellent for treating other infections, such as bronchitis, tonsillitis, strep throat, urinary tract infections, and tooth and gum infections. Echinacea is also useful for helping the immune system fight fungal infections, such as candidiasis. In addition, echinacea is commonly used to treat wounds, burns, bites, stings, and such skin conditions as abscesses, boils, impetigo, herpes, and eczema. Because of its anti-inflammatory effects, echinacea may be helpful for relieving the symptoms of rheumatoid arthritis. And echinacea can help in chronic allergic conditions, such as hay fever, food allergies, and environmental sensitivity.

Infectious diseases respond particularly well to echinacea. This is probably because these diseases are normally dealt with by macrophages, the large white blood cells that devour invading microorganisms. Echinacea is especially effective at stimulating macrophage activity.

Q. Does echinacea have any harmful side effects?

A. A number of laboratory studies have been performed on echinacea using many times the therapeutic dose given to humans, with no toxic side effects. However, the German Commission E, the German authority on herbal remedies, cautions that echinacea should not be used by people who are susceptible to allergic reactions, especially to the *Compositae* (daisy) family. If you have never taken echinacea, begin with a low dose for a couple of days to rule out any individual sensitivity to the herb. For example, try taking ten drops of echinacea liquid extract two times a day and gradually increase the dosage until you are taking the full amount, generally recommended as one dropperful (approximately one-half teaspoon) three times a day.

The most common side effect that can occur with echinacea is caused by taking liquid echinacea extract. The undiluted extract is very strong. Some people report a burning sensation in the back of the throat when they take undiluted echinacea. Others experience a transient tingling sensation on the tongue, and some experience a feeling of nausea associated with the increased salivation that echinacea causes. While unpleasant, none of these symptoms are harmful, and all can be avoided by diluting echinacea extract in a small amount of warm water or by taking echinacea in capsules or tablets.

Q. Can I take echinacea to prevent a cold or flu?

A. Most definitely, yes! In fact, using echinacea to prevent a cold or flu may be the best way to use it. Nipping any infection in the bud is the most assured way of avoiding a more serious illness, so it's always a good idea to take echinacea at the very first sign of a cold or flu, such as a scratchy throat, running nose, or sneezing. I've learned that fatigue is a signal from my body that my immune system is compromised, and I immediately start taking echinacea.

Preventing the infection in the first place is an even better strategy. I use echinacea when I observe others around me getting sick, especially family, friends, and other people that I'm in close contact with. Viruses are spread either through the air or by direct contact. They travel in saliva droplets when an infected person coughs or sneezes, and they also live on doorknobs, telephones, and other surfaces that an infected person has touched. All it takes is for you to touch your nose or eyes, and the virus has found its pathway into your body, where it can multiply and make you sick. Echinacea is completely safe, and it only takes a minute to take a dose of this immune-boosting herb. To prevent illness, take one dropperful of extract in a glass of water or two capsules or tablets three or four times a day.

Q. Will echinacea help me recover faster if I've come down with a cold or flu?

A. It certainly appears that echinacea helps the immune system overcome a cold or flu virus more quickly. I've used echinacea many times to short-circuit a cold or flu, and I've witnessed my family and friends become converts to echinacea once they've tried it for treating a cold or flu. Much of echinacea's popularity has spread in just such a way—through anecdotal, rather than scientific, evidence. But there is also good scientific evidence to prove the efficacy of echinacea.

A 1992 German research study published in the

respected German scientific journal *Zeitschrift fur Phytotherapie* evaluated the effects of echinacea on colds and flu. The study involved 180 male and female subjects between 18 and 60 years of age and was a double-blind, controlled study (this means that half of the subjects were given an extract of echinacea, and half were given a placebo, and neither group nor the researchers knew which group received which until the end). The researchers found that echinacea both relieved cold and flu symptoms and shortened the duration of the illness. In addition, the researchers discovered that while two droppersful daily of echinacea had some effect, four droppersful daily provided a significant reduction in cold symptoms.

Other studies have reported similar positive results. The Swiss medical journal *Schweizerische Zeitschrift fur Ganzheits Medizin* published a study in 1998 showing that tablets of *Echinacea purpurea* were effective against the common cold. At the University Hospital in Uppsala, Sweden, doctors gave 119 patients echinacea or a placebo at a dose of two tablets three times a day for eight days. Of the patients taking echinacea, more than three-fourths reported relief from symptoms such as sore throat, fever, nasal congestion, and cough. In comparison with the placebo, echinacea was found to be twice as effective in relieving symptoms.

Here's an interesting fact that attests to the popularity and efficacy of echinacea. In 1994 alone, echinacea was prescribed for treating the common cold more than 2.5 million times by German physicians and pharmacists.

Q. I get sick a lot. Can I take echinacea to strengthen my overall immunity?

A. This raises a question that is being asked by herbalists, health practitioners, and researchers: Is echinacea primarily an immune stimulant, or can it also be used as an immune tonic? First, it's important to understand the difference between a stimulant and a tonic: A stimulant revs up the immune system, prodding it into action, while a tonic rebuilds and strengthens the foundation of the immune system. Some practitioners and researchers have proposed that because echinacea acts as an immune stimulant, it should not be used for long periods of time because it is not healthy to stimulate the immune system all of the time. They also believe that echinacea should not be used for treating health problems where immune stimulation is inappropriate—for example, in multiple sclerosis, leukemia, collagen disorders, tuberculosis, autoimmune disorders such as rheumatoid arthritis, and

HIV infection and AIDS because the immune system is either already overreactive or not functioning properly. But other researchers believe that echinacea research has been misinterpreted, and that echinacea is best viewed as an immunomodulator, rather than as an immunostimulant.

Q. What is an immunomodulator?

A. Simply put, an immunomodulator is a substance that helps the immune system adapt to changing conditions and thus function more efficiently and effectively. For example, echinacea is well-known for improving macrophage activity. By helping the immune system eliminate the trouble-causing invaders, echinacea helps to bring the body back into balance.

Q. How does this relate to autoimmune diseases?

A. Although the German Commission E stated in 1992 that, in principle, echinacea should not be used by those with autoimmune diseases, there are no clinical studies that show any adverse effects from the use of echinacea in treating these conditions. Immune function is very complex, and some researchers and clinicians are proposing that echinacea is not only safe, but probably beneficial in the treatment of autoimmune disorders. One prominent theory is that autoimmune diseases are initiated by an inappropriate response of the immune system to infectious microorganisms. In line with this theory, echinacea would be helpful in the treatment of autoimmune diseases because it is so effective at enhancing immune response to infectious microorganisms. As a further argument in favor of echinacea, clinicians point out that echinacea has a long history of use as a treatment for autoimmune disorders, such as rheumatoid arthritis. If you suffer from an autoimmune disease and are interested in trying echinacea, it's a good idea to check with your health-care practitioner for guidance.

Q. How does echinacea help in alleviating arthritis?

A. Echinacea has traditionally been used for treating inflammatory diseases such as arthritis, and scientific studies have shown that it reduces inflammation and stimulates the regeneration of healthy tissue. It does this by inhibiting *hyaluronidase*, an enzyme secreted by microorganisms that breaks down *hyaluronic acid*, a primary component of the *ground substance* (sort of an intracellular glue) that holds body cells together. Echinacea also enhances the activity of *fibroblasts*, the cells that produce ground substance. When treating a chronic inflammatory condition such as arthritis, clinical herbalists generally recommend taking echinacea for at least three months and up to nine months at a time. Arthritis, particularly rheumatoid arthritis, is a complex disease and is best addressed with the help of a holistically oriented health practitioner. Many factors need to be taken into consideration, including the identification and elimination of food allergens (the most common allergens are wheat, corn, dairy products, beef, and foods from the nightshade family—tomatoes, potatoes, peppers, and eggplant). Foods that are particularly beneficial for arthritis include fresh fruits and vegetables, which are excellent sources of antioxidants, and foods rich in anti-inflammatory omega-3 fatty acids, such as cold-water fish (salmon, sardines, and mackerel) and flaxseeds or flaxseed oil. Bromelain (an enzyme from pineapple) taken between meals reduces inflammation, and the herbs turmeric and ginger are both powerful anti-inflammatories and can be used in cooking or taken as supplements.

3.

The Healing Properties of Goldenseal

Goldenseal has a long history of use as an infection-fighting herb. Now, more than ever, we need safe alternatives to pharmaceutical antibiotics. In this chapter, you'll learn about the powerful antimicrobial effects of goldenseal, and the research that supports the use of goldenseal as a natural antibiotic.

Q. What is goldenseal?

A. Goldenseal (*Hydrastis canadensis*) is a perennial herb native to rich, moist woodlands in eastern North America. It is a small, hairy-stemmed plant with lobed leaves and has small greenish-white petalless flowers for one week in the spring and

fleshy red berries in July or August. The knotty
rhizome (rootlike stem) has yellow-brown bark and
a bright yellow interior. Medicinally, the rhizome
and root are the most valuable parts of goldenseal.
It takes from three to five years for the roots to
mature to a size that can be harvested. Goldenseal
was once abundant in the eastern forests of the
United States, but the native populations have been
seriously depleted because of overharvesting. Fortunately, this valuable healing plant is now being
cultivated for medicinal use.

Q. Why should I be interested in goldenseal?

A. Goldenseal is a potent antimicrobial that kills
trouble-causing microorganisms, such as bacteria,
fungi, and protozoa. It effectively combats a variety
of infectious diseases that are often treated with
antibiotics, but without the harmful side effects of
pharmaceutical drugs. If you have any type of bacterial or parasitic infection, goldenseal is probably
the best herb you can use. It fights bronchial and
sinus infections; strep throat; urinary tract infections; and skin, eye, and gum infections. Goldenseal
is often paired with echinacea in formulas for treating infectious diseases and strengthening immune

function because the two herbs work well together to combat a wide range of harmful microorganisms.

Q. How does goldenseal work?

A. Berberine, the compound that gives goldenseal root its yellow color, is also responsible for many of the herb's medicinal properties. Berberine has potent antibacterial properties, and has been shown to be effective against a wide variety of bacteria, fungi, and protozoa, including *Staphylococcus* species, *Chlamydia* species, *Escherichia coli*, *Salmonella typhi*, *Giardia lamblia*, and *Candida albicans*. Berberine also improves blood flow to the spleen, the lymphatic organ that filters the blood and releases natural chemicals that stimulate the immune system. In addition, berberine improves immune function by enhancing the activity of the macrophages, the white blood cells that devour cells infected with bacteria, viruses, and cancer.

The bitter components of berberine stimulate bile flow, which improves liver and gallbladder function and eases digestive upsets. Goldenseal also has powerful astringent action, which helps to dry up excess mucus, and anti-inflammatory action, which soothes irritated mucous membranes throughout the body.

Q. How long has goldenseal been used as a healing herb?

A. As with echinacea, goldenseal was commonly used by Native Americans, including the Cherokee, Comanche, Iroquois, and Micmac. They called it yellow root, and used the intense yellow juice from the root as a dye and skin stain. They also considered goldenseal to be a valuable medicinal plant and used it to treat wounds and skin infections, diarrhea, upset stomach, eye infections, fever, sore throats, and cancer, and to help women recover from childbirth. In the early nineteenth century, goldenseal was made popular by Samuel Thomson, the founder of Thomsonian herbal medicine. He gave goldenseal its name, and used it extensively as an antiseptic. The Eclectic physician John King included goldenseal in the first edition of *The Eclectic Dispensatory of the United States of America* (1852), called it *hydrastis*, and recommended it for a wide variety of ailments very similar to the Native American uses.

At that time, goldenseal was an important ingredient in many patent medicine formulas. The popularity of these formulas (Dr. Pierce's Golden Medical Discovery was one of many) increased the demand for goldenseal, and the price for the wildcrafted root soared to one dollar a pound—almost the same price as the popular, expensive ginseng. Goldenseal enjoyed a reputation as a cure-all and longevity tonic, and was referred to as "poor man's ginseng." It was listed in the *U.S. Pharmacopoeia* from 1831 to 1936 as an astringent and antiseptic, until the advent of pharmaceutical antibiotics. The popularity of goldenseal almost led to its demise because of overharvesting of native wild populations.

Q. What are the most common uses for goldenseal?

A. Goldenseal continues to be a popular herb. It is used externally to treat cuts and wounds, boils and other bacterial skin infections, fungal infections such as athlete's foot and ringworm, eczema, acne, eye infections such as conjunctivitis, and hemorrhoids. Internally, goldenseal is used for colds, digestive upsets, and inflamed mucous membranes anywhere in the body. The potent antimicrobial and astringent properties of goldenseal make it especially helpful for treating sore throats, including strep throat, and intestinal infections caused by microbes, such as traveler's diarrhea. Because of its astringency, goldenseal is also helpful for clearing up chronic conditions characterized by excessive mucus, such as sinusitis.

Q. Does goldenseal have any harmful side effects?

A. Goldenseal has a long history of safe use, with no harmful or toxic side effects. However, because of the potential uterine-stimulating properties of berberine, goldenseal should not be used during pregnancy. As with any medicinal herb, if you are using goldenseal for the first time, take a small dose for the first couple of days (ten drops of extract twice a day) to test for individual sensitivity, and gradually increase the amount to the full dosage over several days.

Some researchers caution against the use of goldenseal for people who have high blood pressure. While berberine acts to lower blood pressure, another chemical in goldenseal called hydrastine may raise blood pressure. To err on the side of safety, consult with your health-care practitioner before using goldenseal if you have high blood pressure, heart disease, or a history of stroke.

Q. Is it true that goldenseal is sometimes adultered with other herbs?

A. Unfortunately, that has been true. Because of goldenseal's popularity and high cost, adulteration has been a problem almost from the beginning. One herb that has commonly been substituted for goldenseal is bloodroot (*Sanguinaria canadensis*). Bloodroot is a powerful laxative and in high doses can cause dizziness, vomiting, and purging. You can avoid the problem of adulteration by purchasing goldenseal from reputable herb companies. I recommend buying only goldenseal products that are organically grown. This avoids both the problem of adulteration and the continuing problem of over-harvesting, which threatens to eradicate wild populations of goldenseal.

Q. Would you tell me more about the antibiotic properties of goldenseal?

A. In research and clinical studies, goldenseal has been proven effective at killing a variety of bacteria, fungi, and protozoa. But goldenseal has more than direct antibiotic, or microbe-killing properties. The primary ingredient, berberine, also has other actions that prevent infection, which may be more effective than just antibiotic activity alone. Berberine stimulates immune function, and has been shown to prevent microbes from adhering to host cells. In one study, berberine was shown to be effective in inhibiting the adherence of group A streptococci to host cells. This supports the traditional use of goldenseal in the treatment of strep throat. Goldenseal is also preferable to pharmaceutical antibiotics because it does not disrupt the normal healthy intestinal flora. In fact, berberine is excellent for inhibiting the overgrowth of *Candida albicans*, which often occurs with antibiotic use.

Q. Can goldenseal help protect against intestinal microbes?

A. It definitely can. In a number of clinical studies, berberine has been shown to be very effective in the treatment of acute diarrhea caused by *Giardia lamblia* (the organism that causes giardiasis), *Escherichia coli* (the organism that causes traveler's diarrhea), *Salmonella paratyphi* (one of the organisms that causes food poisoning), and *Vibrio cholerae* (the organism that causes cholera). In fact, berberine appears to be at least as effective as pharmaceutical antibiotics in treating most gastrointestinal infections.

In one study of sixty-five children under the age of five with diarrhea caused by *Escherichia coli*, *Salmonella*, and a variety of other infectious microorganisms, treatment with berberine was found to be more effective than treatment with standard antibiotics. In another study of 200 adults suffering from acute diarrhea, the subjects were given standard antibiotic treatment, but some were also given an extract of berberine. Those who were given berberine recovered more quickly.

According to Michael Murray, N.D., a prominent naturopathic physician and coauthor of *Encyclopedia of Natural Medicine*, much of the effectiveness of berberine can be attributed to its direct antimicrobial activity. In addition, it blocks the effects of the toxins produced by certain infectious bacteria, such as those that cause traveler's diarrhea and cholera. While berberine has been shown to be very effective in treating diarrhea, Murray cautions that because infectious diarrhea is potentially life-threatening, the best approach may be to use standard antibiotic therapy along with goldenseal, especially for diseases such as cholera.

Q. How does goldenseal improve digestive function?

A. Goldenseal has traditionally been used as a "digestive bitter," an herb that improves digestion by stimulating liver and gallbladder function.

Clinical studies have shown that berberine stimulates the secretion of bile, a digestive fluid secreted by the liver and stored in the gallbladder that aids in the digestion and absorption of fats. In one study, 225 patients with chronic inflammation of the gallbladder were given berberine three times daily before meals. Within twenty-four to forty-eight hours, their symptoms had disappeared, and tests showed improvement in gallbladder function.

4.

How to Use Echinacea and Goldenseal Effectively

To use echinacea and goldenseal effectively, it helps to have some basic guidelines. This chapter explains when to take the herbs, how much to take, how much to give to a child, and when to use an echinacea-goldenseal combination product.

Q. How much echinacea should I take?

A. The standard recommendation for taking echinacea is to take one dropperful (approximately one-half teaspoon) of liquid extract or two capsules or tablets three times a day. However, some practitioners recommend taking echinacea in more frequent doses when treating an acute infection. This is thought to be more effective because it saturates the cells with echinacea.

Q. How much echinacea should I take if I have an acute infection?

A. Herbalist and echinacea expert Christopher Hobbs, L.Ac., recommends taking 1 or 2 droppersful (one-half to 1 teaspoon) or 3 to 4 capsules every 2 hours for up to 10 days for treating active infections such as colds, flus, bronchitis, and other upper respiratory tract infections; urinary tract infections; and boils and abscesses. Follow this intensive dose therapy with the standard recommended dose therapy given above.

Q. If I want to take echinacea as a tonic to strengthen my immunity, how should I take it?

A. In general, a tonic dose of an herb is a smaller amount than would be used for treating an acute condition, such as an infection. Tonic doses of herbs are also taken over a longer period of time, usually at least three months, to exert their building and restorative effects. Echinacea expert Christopher Hobbs, L.Ac., recommends taking 10 drops of liquid echinacea extract or 2 capsules once a day for up to nine months to strengthen immune function.

Q. I've heard that if I take echinacea for more than a week at a time, it loses its effectiveness.

A. This is an area of much controversy among herbalists, researchers, and health practitioners. Many practitioners recommend that echinacea be taken in cycles—for example, ten days on and four days off, or two weeks on and two weeks off. This is based on the interpretation of a study that seemed to indicate that using echinacea continuously causes the immune system to get accustomed to the herb and, therefore, no longer responsive to the stimulation provided by echinacea.

Recently, however, some researchers and clinicians have pointed out that the study was misinterpreted, and that echinacea *does not* lose its effectiveness, even when used over long periods of time. In fact, one study showed that the effects of echinacea on the immune system were even greater after ten weeks of continual usage than after two weeks.

It seems that whether you choose to use echinacea in cycles or continuously, it will still have a potent immune-enhancing effect. If you are treating a condition of chronic immune deficiency, consult your health-care practitioner for guidance in using echinacea.

Q. How much goldenseal should I take?

A. The standard recommended dose for goldenseal is 1 to 2 droppersful (about one-half to 1 teaspoon) of fluid extract or 2 to 4 capsules 3 times a day. If you are treating an acute infection and taking a combination echinacea-goldenseal product, follow the recommendations given above for treating acute infections.

Q. Can I take goldenseal as a tonic herb to strengthen my immune system?

A. While goldenseal does have some immune-enhancing effects, its primary value lies in its antimicrobial action. Therefore, goldenseal is best used for treating acute infections, while echinacea is appropriate for long-term immune strengthening. There are times when it may be helpful to take goldenseal for longer than the ten days recommended for acute infections, for example, when treating a deep-seated fungal infection, such as candidiasis. It can take one month or longer for goldenseal to effectively knock back the *Candida albicans* organism.

Q. Does goldenseal wipe out beneficial intestinal flora?

A. While goldenseal does eradicate unfriendly, disease-causing microorganisms, there is no indication that it disrupts healthy intestinal bacteria.

Q. Is it better to take echinacea and goldenseal with meals?

A. It doesn't really matter too much. As a rule of thumb, many herbalists recommend taking liquid extracts in a small amount of warm water about fifteen minutes before meals because the herbs are quickly absorbed into the bloodstream on an empty stomach. Capsules and tablets are usually best taken after meals to reduce the possibility of stomach upset. One effect of echinacea extract is that when it comes into contact with the tongue, it stimulates saliva flow, which for some people is an unpleasant sensation. Undiluted goldenseal extract can cause irritation of the mucous membranes in the throat. Always dilute liquid extracts, and if you are especially sensitive, take extracts with meals.

Q. How much echinacea should I give to a child?

A. Echinacea is an excellent, safe herb to give to children. Again, while an allergic reaction is extremely unlikely, if you've never given a child echinacea before, test for individual sensitivity by giving just a few drops twice a day for a couple of days, gradually increasing the dosage to the full amount over several days. According to Joseph Pizzorno, N.D., president of Bastyr College, one-half the adult dosage is appropriate for children under the age of six (about one-quarter teaspoon three times a day) and the full adult dosage (about one-half teaspoon three times a day) can be given to children over the age of six. If a child balks at the slightly bitter taste of echinacea, try diluting the tincture in a small amount of juice to disguise the flavor. Echinacea extracts made especially for children are also available, and are sweetened with vegetable glycerin and fruit flavors.

Q. Why does echinacea extract make my tongue numb?

A. First of all, be reassured that this is not a harmful reaction. Echinacea contains natural chemicals called alkylamides, which have a mild anesthetic effect and cause a tingling sensation on the tongue. Alkylamides are primarily concentrated in echinacea roots, and occur in higher concentration in *E. angustifolia* than in *E. purpurea* or *E. pallida*.

Q. The label on my bottle of herbal extract says to dilute the extract in water. Why?

A. Herbal extracts are highly concentrated—one dropperful is equivalent to one cup of tea. While some people take herbal extracts "straight," most people find that diluting the extract in water (or juice or tea) makes the herb easier to take. This is especially true for strong-tasting herbs such as echinacea or goldenseal. Natural chemical constituents in echinacea stimulate salivation, which can last for several minutes and may cause a feeling of nausea for some people. Undiluted goldenseal extract can irritate the mucous membranes of the throat and cause a burning sensation. While these are not harmful effects, they are also not pleasant. Diluting the extract in a small amount of liquid takes care of the problem.

Another reason to dilute herbal extracts is that alcohol-based herbal extracts contain a large percentage of alcohol. If you want to minimize the alcohol content of the extract, pour a small amount (about one-quarter cup) of boiling water over the herb dosage to evaporate off most of the alcohol.

Q. Why are echinacea and goldenseal often combined in herbal products?

A. Echinacea and goldenseal both enhance immune activity, and both have antimicrobial properties. However, goldenseal has much more powerful antimicrobial properties and is effective against a wide range of infectious microorganisms. Echinacea has more potent immune-stimulating properties. The combination of echinacea and goldenseal is excellent for treating a variety of infectious diseases. For example, you can take only echinacea for a cold or flu, but by also taking goldenseal, you have the added benefit of potent antibacterial action, which helps to fight off any secondary bacterial infection that could lead to bronchitis or pneumonia.

Q. When should I take an echinacea-goldenseal combination instead of just echinacea?

A. Basically, you can take an echinacea-goldenseal combination product for any infectious disease. Taking both is especially indicated when treating any type of infection that may be caused by bacteria, fungi, or protozoa, such as strep throat, bronchial infections, sinusitis, urinary tract infections, candidiasis, and gastrointestinal tract infections.

Q. Why would I want to use echinacea and goldenseal to treat an infection when antibiotics work so well?

A. It's true that pharmaceutical antibiotics are miracle drugs. They have saved countless lives, and there are times when they are definitely necessary. But because antibiotics have been overprescribed and used inappropriately, a whole new health crisis has emerged. In recent years, scientists and doctors have found mutant strains of bacteria that are resistant to antibiotics. Diseases that were thought to be eradicated, such as tuberculosis, are reappearing— but are no longer responding to the antibiotics that once so easily kept them under control. In some cases, the antibiotics needed to kill the super germs are virtually as dangerous as the disease.

There are other problems associated with the use of antibiotics. Every time you take an antibiotic, you are killing not only the problem-causing microbes, but you are also killing the friendly bacteria that inhabit your intestinal tract. These friendly bacteria are essential for your good health. Among other tasks, they aid digestion and intestinal function, help in the complex task of detoxification, and prevent the overgrowth of microorganisms that cause genitourinary tract infections. A disrupted intestinal ecology can cause many health problems, including digestive disturbances, elevated cholesterol levels, yeast infections, arthritis, and premenstrual and menopausal difficulties.

While echinacea and goldenseal have antibiotic properties, they do not eradicate friendly bacteria in the body. Echinacea primarily strengthens your immune system, which ultimately is your best defense against invaders anyway. The world is teeming with microorganisms, and a lot of them are unfriendly. We've learned the hard way that it's not possible, nor is it desirable, to try to eradicate them all. The answer is not to try to come up with ever more potent antibiotics. A more holistic and healthy approach is to focus on improving your natural defenses.

Q. How much echinacea should I take if I've already got a cold or flu?

A. Some health practitioners recommend the same dosage necessary for preventing a cold or flu: 1 dropperful of liquid extract or 2 capsules or tablets 3 or 4 times a day. Others suggest taking a lot more, with the idea of saturating the body tissues with echinacea and keeping immune response highly activated. For example, herbalist Christopher Hobbs, L.Ac., recommends taking 1 to 2 droppersful (approximately one-half to 1 teaspoon) or 3 to 4 capsules of echinacea every 2 hours for up to 10 days at a time to fight off an infection.

Q. Should I take goldenseal to combat a cold or flu?

A. It's not a bad idea, because upper respiratory infections are often followed by a secondary bacterial infection (such as bronchitis) that takes hold when resistance is low. The powerful antibacterial properties of goldenseal help to fight off any trouble-causing bacteria. In addition, the astringent action of goldenseal is helpful for drying up the excessive mucus secretions that accompany a cold or flu. Many formulas designed for treating colds and flus combine echinacea with goldenseal for these reasons.

Q. What else can I do to help my body recover from a cold or flu?

A. First of all, get lots of rest. The immune system functions optimally with plenty of rest, and is most active during sleep. Avoid all sweets, which depress immune function, and eat light, nourishing foods, such as soups and lightly cooked vegetables. Drink plenty of fluids to thin mucus congestion. Take 1,000 mg or more of vitamin C daily, which has been shown to shorten the duration of colds. Zinc lozenges (supplying between 15 and 25 mg of zinc) help to prevent the virus from replicating. Take two lozenges initially, followed by one lozenge every two hours to a maximum of 10 lozenges per day for up to seven days.

Q. Can echinacea and goldenseal be used for treating serious respiratory illnesses, such as bronchitis or pneumonia?

A. Bronchitis and pneumonia are potentially serious illnesses that most often follow a bout with the flu or a cold. Bronchitis is caused by irritation or infection of the lining of the bronchial tubes, the airways that lead from the windpipe to the lungs. Symptoms include a persistent, mucus-producing cough and a feeling of breathlessness. Pneumonia is an infection of one or both lungs, most often caused by a virus but sometimes caused by bacteria. Symptoms of pneumonia include fever, chills, chest pain, breathlessness, and coughing that produces green, yellow, or blood-tinged mucus.

Because bronchitis and pneumonia may be caused by bacteria, antibiotics are almost always prescribed by conventional medical practitioners. If you suspect either of these diseases, it's essential to consult with your health-care practitioner. Both bronchitis and pneumonia can be life-threatening diseases for someone who is elderly or immune-compromised. However, note that antibiotics are of absolutely no use in treating virus-caused bronchitis or pneumonia. Echinacea is an excellent immune-strengthening herb for helping the body overcome the infection, and goldenseal helps to fight bacteria that may be causing the infection.

Q. What else can I do to help my body recover from a serious respiratory illness?

A. Rest is essential for recovery from bronchitis or pneumonia. Drink plenty of fluids to thin mucus secretions, especially herbal teas, such as those made with ginger, which help to relieve congestion. Eat warm, nourishing foods, such as soups, and eat a couple cloves of chopped raw garlic daily for its powerful antibacterial and antiviral properties.

To relieve chest congestion and stimulate the release of mucus, massage the upper back and chest with a mentholated chest rub. Buy herbal cough syrups that contain expectorants such as licorice (*Glycyrrhize glabra*), wild cherry bark (*Prunus spp.*), and horehound (*Marrubium vulgare*) to help the lungs expel mucus. Joseph Pizzorno, N.D., also recommends the technique of postural drainage to help rid the lungs of excess mucus. Apply a hot-water bottle to the chest for twenty minutes, and then lie face down on the bed with the top half of the body from the waist down hanging off of the bed, supporting the upper body with the forearms. Stay in this position for at least five minutes, and attempt to clear the lungs by coughing up mucus.

Q. Should I use echinacea or goldenseal for treating a sore throat?

A. It's probably best to use both. Echinacea and goldenseal both bolster the immune system to overcome the infection, and goldenseal has the added benefit of acting as a powerful antibiotic in the case of a bacterial infection. In addition, goldenseal has anti-inflammatory and astringent effects that constrict swollen tissues. A severe sore throat, especially one without cold symptoms and accompanied by a fever higher than 101 degrees, white spots on the tonsils, or swollen glands, should be evaluated by a health-care practitioner to rule out strep throat.

Strep throat is a potentially serious illness that

can cause rheumatic fever and kidney damage. It is almost always treated with antibiotics, even though recent studies show that recovery is similar whether antibiotics are taken or not. Naturopathic physicians Joseph Pizzorno and Michael Murray suggest that antibiotics be reserved for people who are suffering from a severe infection, those who have a prior history of rheumatic fever or strep-induced kidney disease, or those who have not responded within one week to natural therapies.

Improving the strength of the immune system with echinacea and goldenseal helps the body to naturally fight off the strep organism. Goldenseal has been proven effective at killing streptococci, and also prevents the strep bacteria from adhering to the mucous membranes of the throat. When treating a sore throat, take one-half to 1 teaspoon of echinacea-goldenseal liquid extract or 3 to 4 capsules every two waking hours for up to 10 days.

Q. What else can I do to recover from a sore throat?

A. As with an upper respiratory infection, be sure to drink plenty of fluids to keep mucous membranes hydrated, which helps to make the environment inhospitable for infectious microorganisms.

Hot teas, such as those made with ginger and licorice root, are helpful for soothing inflamed throat tissues. Gargle with warm salt water every couple of hours to temporarily relieve pain, using one-half tablespoon of salt dissolved in one cup of water as warm as you can tolerate. For extra antimicrobial and anti-inflammatory support, add one dropperful of goldenseal extract to the gargle. Supplements that help to strengthen immune function include at least 1,000 mg of vitamin C daily, and one 15- to 25-mg zinc lozenge every two hours, for a maximum of 10 lozenges a day for seven days.

Q. Can I use goldenseal to treat diarrhea?

A. Goldenseal is an excellent remedy for diarrhea, both because its potent antibacterial properties have been proven to kill the microorganisms that cause infectious diarrhea (such as traveler's diarrhea) and because the astringent effects of goldenseal soothe the irritated mucous membranes of the gastrointestinal tract. Michael Murray, N.D., suggests taking goldenseal as a preventive measure before traveling to an underdeveloped country or an area known to have poor water quality or sanitation. He recommends taking goldenseal for the duration of the trip, as well as one week prior to leaving and one week after returning. A standard dose of goldenseal is one-half to 1 teaspoon of liquid extract or 3 to 4 capsules three times a day.

Note that any case of diarrhea that does not resolve within a few days (or forty-eight hours in a child under the age of three) should be evaluated by a health-care practitioner.

Q. What else should I do when treating diarrhea?

A. Usually, the biggest problem with acute diarrhea is dehydration from the excessive amounts of fluids lost in frequent bowel movements. Dehydration can quickly become serious in infants, young children, and the elderly. Be sure to increase fluid intake to at least two quarts of water daily. To replenish the essential minerals that diarrhea flushes from the body, drink natural apple juice diluted with an equal amount of water or an electrolyte replacement drink. Eat foods that help to bind loose stools, such as bananas, rice, applesauce, and toast, and avoid foods that may be irritating, such as spicy or fatty foods, coffee, dairy products, and citrus juices.

Q. Can I use echinacea and goldenseal for treating urinary tract infections?

A. Yes, and it's probably preferable to the antibiotics that are commonly prescribed for treating such infections. Most urinary tract infections are caused by the bacteria *Escherichia coli*. These bacteria occur normally in the intestinal tract, and cause infection when they migrate up the urethra and into the bladder. Symptoms of a bladder infection include increased frequency and urgency of urination and burning upon urination. Antibiotics are almost always prescribed for treating urinary tract infections, but antibiotic treatment frequently causes a rebound vaginal yeast infection, and research suggests that antibiotics contribute to recurrent bladder infections.

Echinacea stimulates the immune system to help the body fight the infection, and goldenseal has long been used in treating bladder infections and is especially helpful because of its ability to kill the *E. coli* organism. Take one-half to 1 teaspoon of echinacea-goldenseal liquid extract or 3 to 4 capsules every two waking hours for up to 10 days.

If symptoms do not improve within a couple of days, consult your health-care practitioner. If your symptoms include low- to mid-back pain, fever, or blood in the urine, do not attempt self-treatment.

See your health-care practitioner immediately to
rule out a kidney infection, which can cause serious
damage to the kidneys.

Q. What else should I do to recover from a urinary tract infection?

A. Be sure to drink plenty of fluids, which helps to
flush the infectious microorganisms from the bladder. Infection can only occur if the bacteria can gain
a foothold and multiply. Drink at least two quarts of
liquid daily, avoiding all sweetened drinks. Cranberry juice has been shown to prevent and relieve
urinary tract infections by making the walls of
the bladder slippery and inhospitable to bacteria.
Drink 16 ounces of unsweetened cranberry juice
diluted with an equal amount of unsweetened
apple juice. Because cranberry juice may make the
urine slightly acidic, and goldenseal works best in
an alkaline environment, it's probably best to avoid
cranberry juice, ascorbic acid (vitamin C), and other
acidic foods while using goldenseal. However, if
you are prone to urinary tract infections, you can
drink cranberry juice on a regular basis to prevent
infections.

Q. How can echinacea and goldenseal be used for treating candidiasis?

A. Caused by an overgrowth of the *Candida albicans* yeast in the digestive tract, candidiasis is a complex disorder that requires killing off the trouble-causing fungus and strengthening the immune system at the same time. The *Candida* organism is a normal inhabitant of the digestive tract and the vagina, but it can grow out of control when antibiotics kill off the beneficial intestinal flora that keep it in check. Symptoms include fatigue, depression, irritability, allergies, digestive disturbances, and frequent vaginal yeast and bladder infections.

The *Candida albicans* organism produces a large number of toxins that stress the immune system, making it difficult for normal immune mechanisms to overcome the fungal overgrowth. Echinacea bolsters the immune system and can help to restore healthy immune function. Goldenseal has direct antifungal activity and has been proven to be effective at killing the *Candida* organism. Take one-half to 1 teaspoon of echinacea-goldenseal liquid extract or 3 to 4 capsules three times daily for one to three months.

Q. What else can I do to help my body recover from candidiasis?

A. The most effective way to control *Candida albicans* overgrowth is to bring the body back into balance so that it naturally keeps the organism in check. Avoid foods that promote *Candida* overgrowth, such as sugar and large amounts of honey, maple syrup, and fruit juice; dairy products; foods containing large amounts of yeasts or molds, such as alcohol, dried fruits, and peanuts; and food allergens. Improving digestion with the use of digestive enzymes or preparations of herbal digestive bitters is often helpful, and restoring healthy intestinal flora is essential for keeping the *Candida* organism under control. Take supplements of *Lactobacillus acidophilus* and *Bifidobacteria bifidum* daily for one month or longer to repopulate the intestinal tract with beneficial organisms. To help fight the overgrowth of *Candida*, eat one or two cloves of raw garlic daily, which has potent antifungal properties.

Q. How is echinacea used externally?

A. Echinacea is excellent for external use as a general antiseptic and antimicrobial. It fights a wide variety of microorganisms, and in liquid extract form, makes an effective skin wash for preventing and treating external infections. You can make a simple antiseptic wash by diluting liquid echinacea extract with an equal amount of water. Apply with a sterile cotton ball, or keep the mixture in a small spray bottle for easy application to cuts and wounds.

For infected cuts, wounds, or boils, apply echinacea extract full strength. Soak a sterile cotton pad with liquid echinacea and bandage it to the affected area. Keep the dressing moist, and apply a fresh cotton pad several times a day. In addition, take echinacea internally to help fight the infection, one-half to one teaspoon of liquid extract or 3 to 4 capsules three times a day until the infection is gone. Use full-strength echinacea also for insect bites and stings, impetigo, and herpes. For treating mouth and gum infections and sore throats, gargle with one-half cup of warm water mixed with one dropperful of echinacea extract, and swallow the mixture. Repeat three to four times a day. Also apply echinacea full-strength with a cotton swab to canker sores or inflamed gums.

Q. How is goldenseal used externally?

A. Goldenseal is extremely useful for a wide variety of external infections. A simple tea can be made of the powdered herb by pouring one cup of boiling water over one teaspoon of powdered goldenseal. Goldenseal can be bought in bulk, or it is readily available in capsules that can be opened and measured. Steep the herb for fifteen minutes, and then strain through a coffee filter. Use caution when working with goldenseal—it stains anything it touches yellow. (Remember that the Native Americans used goldenseal as a dye!) If you choose, you can also use a liquid extract of goldenseal by adding one dropperful of extract to one cup of warm water.

Use the goldenseal tea as a mouthwash for treating gum inflammation or canker sores, as an eye wash for soothing conjuctivitis or blepharitis, or as a skin wash for treating cuts, wounds, and fungal infections, such as athlete's foot and ringworm. The tea can also be used as a douche for vaginal infections. To calm itching from eczema, insect bites, or hemorrhoids, dilute one-half dropperful of goldenseal extract in one-half cup of distilled witch hazel and apply to the affected area.

5.

How to Choose Echinacea and Goldenseal Products

Echinacea and goldenseal are top-selling herbs, and the vast assortment of products containing one or both of these herbs attests to their popularity. Choosing among the many products on the market can be confusing. In this chapter, you will learn how to identify good-quality products and understand the differences among the various herbal formulations. Armed with this information, you will be able to make an informed decision that will help you to choose a product that best meets your needs.

Q. What part of the echinacea plant has medicinal properties?

A. All parts of the echinacea plant—the flowers

(which contain the seed heads), leaves, stems, and roots—have medicinal properties, although the roots and seeds are considered to have the most powerful benefits. In addition, all varieties of echinacea appear to have immune-enhancing properties, although they differ in their chemical makeup. The varieties of echinacea commonly used in commercial preparations are *Echinacea purpurea*, *Echinacea angustifolia*, and *Echinacea pallida*.

The above-ground parts of the plant (the flower heads, leaves, and stems) are harvested when the plant is blooming, generally in the late summer. The roots are harvested in the late fall from plants that are three to four years old. According to echinacea expert Christopher Hobbs, L.Ac., herbalists and herbal manufacturers agree that echinacea products should contain at least one part of or a combination of the root, leaf, and flower of *E. purpurea* plus the root of *E. angustifolia*. While *E. pallida* is sometimes included in echinacea preparations, it has not been studied as extensively as *E. purpurea* and *E. angustifolia*.

Q. Are products made from fresh echinacea better than those made from the dried plant?

A. The majority of scientific and clinical studies on echinacea have used a German product made from the freshly pressed juice of *Echinacea purpurea* flowering plant tops stabilized with alcohol (this preparation is known as a "succus"). This does not mean that other types of echinacea preparations are not just as valuable. There are many different types of echinacea products on the market, including liquid-extract tinctures made with grain alcohol or glycerin and water; capsules or tablets of freeze-dried extracts or simple herb powders; and *E. purpurea* succus.

A simple guideline is to remember that an herbal preparation can only be as potent as the raw plant material that goes into it. The fresher the plant, the more likely it is to contain a high concentration of active ingredients. Therefore, when buying echinacea products, look for those made from fresh plants. Read product labels—they will clearly state if fresh echinacea was used.

Q. What part of the goldenseal plant has medicinal properties?

A. The root and rhizome of goldenseal contain the active medicinal properties. They contain a high concentration of berberine, which has been identified as the primary healing constituent. It takes at least three years for a goldenseal root to be large enough to harvest.

Q. Are products made from fresh goldenseal better than those made from the dried plant?

A. There are many different types of goldenseal preparations on the market, including liquid extracts made with grain alcohol or glycerin and water, and capsules or tablets of freeze-dried extracts or simple herb powders. As with echinacea, a simple guideline to remember is that an herbal preparation can only be as potent as the raw plant material that it is made from. The fresher the plant, the more likely it is to contain a high concentration of active ingredients. Therefore, when buying any goldenseal preparation, look for one made from fresh plants. If you read the product label, it will tell you if fresh goldenseal was used.

Q. What does it mean when the manufacturer says the herb was wildcrafted?

A. A wildcrafted herb is one that has been harvested from its natural habitat. For centuries, herbs have been wildcrafted from native populations of plants. But with the increasing interest in herbal medicine, wild plant populations are being seriously threatened by overharvesting. This is especially true for popular herbs such as echinacea and goldenseal. Most herbalists and botanists agree that echinacea and goldenseal populations cannot sustain current wildcrafting demands. Fortunately, there is no need to wildcraft either one. Goldenseal and the three varieties of echinacea used medicinally—*E. purpurea*, *E. angustifolia*, and *E. pallida*—can all be cultivated. In fact, most of the world's supply of *E. purpurea* is currently cultivated.

Q. What does it mean when the manufacturer says the herb was organically grown?

A. Organically grown herbs are those grown without the use of synthetic chemicals, such as fertilizers, fungicides, herbicides, and pesticides. In many cases, agricultural chemicals are systemic, which means that they become a part of the plant and are found in any product made from treated plants. These types of chemicals poison not only the plant, but also the soil, the water, and the air. Most, if not all, echinacea and goldenseal products are made from organically grown or wildcrafted herbs. Organically grown echinacea and goldenseal plants are much preferred to wildcrafted plants because of the problem of overharvesting discussed above. In addition, with organically grown plants, you can be assured of exactly what you are getting.

Q. Should I take liquid extracts, tablets, or capsules of echinacea and goldenseal?

A. It's really your choice. The most important consideration is to buy products that are made from fresh echinacea and/or goldenseal and to buy a preparation that you feel comfortable taking. Some people like using liquid extracts, while others prefer the familiarity of capsules or tablets. I prefer liquid extracts of echinacea and goldenseal, but I carry capsules of freeze-dried products when I'm traveling. Be aware that preparations can vary in potency, depending on the quality of the raw plant material, the care taken in the manufacturing process, and how long the product has been sitting on the shelf in the store or at your home. If you try one type of product and don't feel that it helped you, then try another product until you find one that you are satisfied with.

Q. What exactly is a fluid extract, and how is it different from a tincture?

A. The terms are often used interchangeably, but there is a difference between a tincture and a fluid extract. Tinctures are made by steeping the herb in food-grade alcohol, which extracts medicinal properties that are not water-soluble (water-soluble properties are also extracted because water is used along with the alcohol). A fluid extract is basically a concentrated tincture. Concentration methods used by manufacturers include using larger amounts of the herb, steeping the herb for a longer time, and using evaporation or percolation.

Herb books often refer to any alcohol-based liquid extract as a tincture, which can create some confusion. Many herb books give directions for making simple herbal tinctures at home, which basically involves chopping the herb and steeping it in vodka for two or three weeks. What you'll find for sale by herbal product manufacturers are fluid extracts. They have specialized equipment for grinding, pressing, percolating, and otherwise making concentrated extracts.

Q. How much alcohol am I getting when I take a liquid extract or a tincture?

A. If you take three to four doses a day of a liquid extract or tincture (the standard dropperful, or about one-quarter teaspoon), your total alcohol intake is less than one-half teaspoon. You can evaporate off most of the alcohol by pouring one-quarter cup of boiling water over your dosage and letting it cool to room temperature before drinking it.

Q. How long do echinacea and goldenseal preparations retain their potency?

A. It depends on the type of preparation and how it is stored. The most damaging elements to herbal products are heat, light, moisture, and air. This eliminates storage in the bathroom medicine cabinet and the kitchen cupboard above the stove! Liquid extracts are the most stable of all herbal preparations. Because they are preserved in alcohol or glycerin, they have a long shelf life—anywhere from three to five years when stored in a cool, dark place, such as a pantry or a kitchen cupboard away from the stove. Tablets and capsules have a shorter shelf life—up to about six months. They should also be stored in a cool, dark place away from moisture. I generally recommend buying herbs in small quantities to make sure that your supply is always fresh.

Q. Some products are labeled as standardized extracts. What does this mean?

A. Standardized extracts are herbal products that are guaranteed to contain a specified amount of what is currently believed to be the herb's primary active ingredient. Various procedures are used to obtain the specified concentration, including removing what are considered to be unimportant constituents and adding high concentrations of the isolated active ingredient.

As with many herbs, there is controversy as to what is actually the primary active ingredient. In the case of echinacea, some standardized products use echinacoside as a standard measure. However, some studies have shown that this is not the most potent ingredient in echinacea, and it is not even found in *E. purpurea*. Some preparations of the fresh-pressed juice of *E. purpurea* are standardized based upon the ingredient beta-1,2-fructofuranosides. According to echinacea expert Christoper Hobbs, L.Ac., other active ingredients, such as alkylamides, may eventually be used for standardizing products.

Q. Should I buy a standardized extract?

A. Standardized extracts were created out of the need for consistent results in scientific studies. But many herbalists believe that there may be other constituents in a whole herb extract that are just as important. In other words, products made from the whole plant have a greater and more balanced effect than any individual isolated constituent. You may want to try using a whole herb extract, and if you don't get the results you want, try a standardized extract and see if there is any difference in effect.

Q. How can I find a qualified herbalist who will work with me in my use of echinacea and goldenseal?

A. Look for an herbalist who is a professional member of the American Herbalists Guild. Professional members are admitted by peer review and must have three years of clinical experience. Contact the American Herbalists Guild, P.O. Box 70, Roosevelt, UT 84066, phone (435) 722-8434. Many naturopathic physicians also specialize in herbal medicine. To find a naturopathic physician in your area, contact the American Association of Naturopathic Physicians, 2366 Eastlake Avenue, Suite 322, Seattle, WA 98102, phone (206) 323-7610.

Conclusion

By now, you have a good understanding of how echinacea and goldenseal can improve your health. You know how these valuable herbs work to support your natural immunity and fight disease-causing microorganisms, and you know how to use them.

As I mentioned in the Introduction, echinacea and goldenseal are two of my favorite herbs, and I've used and recommended them countless times to treat a wide variety of infections. In more than twenty-five years, I have not taken any pharmaceutical antibiotics, and I credit these two herbs with preventing this need. Both herbs have a long history of safe use, and their soaring popularity is proof that they are meeting a pressing need for safe alternatives to the pharmaceutical antibiotics that we have relied so heavily on, to our detriment.

Use this information wisely to stay healthy, and remember to always consult your health-care practitioner in the case of a serious or lingering infection. I wish you good health!

Glossary

Alkylamide. A fat-soluble constituent of echinacea that has immune-enhancing properties.

Antibody. A protein molecule produced by the B cells that combines with an antigen and disables it.

Antigen. A foreign substance, such as a virus, that provokes an immune response.

Astringent. A substance that causes the constriction of tissue.

Berberine. The primary active ingredient in goldenseal, responsible for the herb's antimicrobial effects.

Complement fractions. Small proteins that circulate in the blood and enhance immune, allergic, and inflammatory reactions.

Echinacoside. Natural chemical compound in echinacea believed to have mild antibiotic activity.

Immunomodulator. A substance that helps the immune system adapt to changing conditions.

Interferon. A protein produced by virus-infected cells that inhibits reproduction of the virus and promotes resistance to further infection.

Interleukin. A protein produced by T cells and macrophages that stimulates the growth and activity of white blood cells.

Leukocyte. A white blood cell that fights infection.

Macrophage. A large white blood cell that engulfs and devours harmful microorganisms and infected and damaged cells.

Natural killer cell. A type of lymphocyte that has the ability to kill a wide range of infectious microorganisms and tumor cells.

Phagocyte. A white blood cell that engulfs and destroys infected and damaged cells.

Polyacetylene. A fat-soluble constituent of echinacea that has immune-enhancing properties.

Polysaccharide. A large, water-soluble, complex sugar molecule believed to cause an immune-stimulating response in echinacea.

References

Bauer R, et al., "Influence of echinacea extracts on phagocytotic activity," *Zeitschrift fur Phytotherapie* 10 (1989): 43–48.

Bone K, "Echinacea. What Makes it Work?" *Alternative Medicine Review*, 2 (6) (1997): 87–93.

Bone K, "Echinacea. When Should It Be Used?" *Alternative Medicine Review* 2 (6) (1997): 451–458.

Braunig B, et al., "*Echinacea Purpureae* Radix for Strengthening the Immune Response in Flu-Like Infections," *Zeitschrift fur Phytotherapie* 13 (1992): 7–13.

Brinkeborn R, et al., "Echinaforce in the treatment of acute colds. Results of a placebo-controlled double-blind study carried out in Sweden," *Schweizerische Zeitschrift fur Ganzheits Medizin* 10 (1998): 26–29.

Castleman M, *The Healing Herbs*. Emmaus, PA: Rodale Press, 1991.

Desai AB, et al., "Berberine in the treatment of diarrhoea," *Indian Pediatr* 8 (1971): 462–465.

Foster S, *Herbal Renaissance*. Salt Lake City, UT: Gibbs-Smith, 1993.

Gupte S, "Use of berberine in the treatment of giardiasis," *Am J Dis Child*, 129 (1975): 866.

Lohmann-Matthes M, et al., "Macrophage activation by plant polysaccharides," *Z Phytother* 10 (2) (1989): 52–59.

Murray M, *The Healing Power of Herbs*. Rocklin, CA: Prima Publishing, 1995.

Murray M and Pizzorno J, *Encyclopedia of Natural Medicine*. Rocklin, CA: Prima Publishing, 1998.

Sabir M, et al., "Study of some pharmacologic actions of berberine," *Indian J Physiol Pharmacol* 15 (1971): 111–132.

Sack RB, et. al., "Berberine inhibits intestinal secretory response of *Vibrio cholerae* toxins and *Escherichia coli* enterotoxins," *Infect Immun* 35 (1982): 471–475.

Sun D, et al., "Berberine sulfate blocks adherence of *Streptococcus pyogenes* to epithelial cells, fibronectin, and hexadecane," *Antimicrob Agents Chemother* 32 (1988): 1370–1374.

Wagner H, "Herbal immunostimulants," *Zeitschrift fur Phytotherapie* 17 (2) (1996): 79–95.

Suggested Readings

Chaitow L. *Antibiotic Crisis: Antibiotic Alternatives*. Hammersmith, London: Thorsons, 1998.

Hobbs C. *Echinacea, The Immune Herb*. Santa Cruz, CA: Botanic Press, 1996.

Huemer RP and Challem J. *The Natural Health Guide to Beating the Supergerms*. New York: Pocket Books, 1997.

McKenna J. *Natural Alternatives to Antibiotics*. Garden City Park, NY: Avery Publishing Group, 1998.

Murray M. and Pizzorno J. *Encyclopedia of Natural Medicine*. Rocklin, CA: Prima Publishing, 1998.

Index